DIET

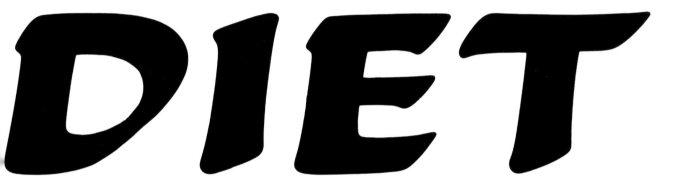

Brian Ward

FRANKLIN WATTS

New York/London/Sydney/Toronto

© Franklin Watts 1991

Franklin Watts, Inc.
387 Park Avenue South
New York, N.Y. 10016

Library of Congress Cataloging-in-Publication Data
Ward, Brian R.
    Diet / Brian Ward.
        p.   cm. — (Health guides)
    Summary: An introduction to the digestive system, focusing on
dietary problems, eating disorders, and ways to maintain a proper
diet.
    ISBN 0-531-14095-4
    1. Nutrition—Juvenile literature.   2. Diet—Juvenile literature.
3. Eating disorders—Juvenile literature.   4. Gastrointestinal
system—Juvenile literature.   [1. Nutrition.   2. Diet.
3. Digestive system.]   I. Title.   II. Series.
QP141.W367   1991   3. Digestion.
613.2—dc20   90-31200
                                                    CIP AC

Illustrations: Simon Roulstone

Photographs: B & C Alexander 21bl; Bubbles/Jenny Woodcock
5t, 11b; Chris Fairclough cover, 4b, 6bl, 6br, 8b, 10t, 10b, 11t, 12t,
13t, 15tr, 16t, 18t, 19b, 20c, 20b, 24b, 26, 27tl, 27tr, 28t, 30b; Chris
Fairclough Colour Library 17b, 19c; with thanks to Gibbs Elida
11c; Susan Griggs Agency/Cornstock 28b; Robert Harding Picture
Library 19t, (F Hache) 25t, 27br; Hutchison Library 16b, 18b, 22b,
29b; with thanks to the Japanese Information Service 14b; Peter
Millard 5bl, 23t; Network (Spartum) 4t, (Barry Lewis) 6t,
(Goldwater) 8t; Rex Features 25b; Frank Spooner Pictures 5br;
Science Photo Library (Carl Schmidt) 9t, (Martin Dohrn) 12b, 21t,
(David Scharf) 20t, (US Dept. of Energy) 21br, (Tektoff, RM/CNRI)
22t, (John Radcliffe Hospital) 27bl; Supersport Photographs/
Eileen Langsley 9bl; ZEFA 15tl, 24t.

Printed in Belgium

CONTENTS

FEELING GOOD

A healthy diet is essential for a healthy body. Our entire body is constructed from the food we eat. To provide for all our needs food must contain the right mixture of nutrients or food substances. Once you understand what your body needs, it is usually quite easy to eat a healthy diet by eating plenty of the foods which contain the most important nutrients, and avoiding some "junk" food.

A healthy diet is particularly important while you are growing rapidly. At this time your body needs extra amounts of some nutrients, to build healthy bones and teeth, for example. Quality and not quantity is the rule for a healthy diet, and most of us eat far more than we really need.

However, a healthy diet is not enough to keep you healthy. You need exercise to keep your body working properly, and to keep you from becoming overweight.

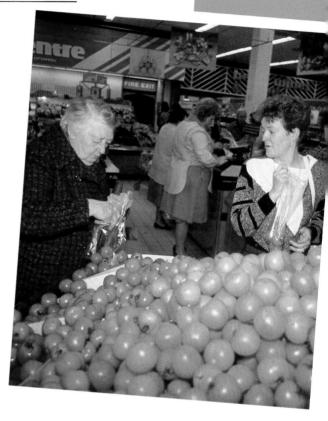

△ We are fortunate in being able to buy a range of foods, which allows us to eat a healthy, mixed diet. If you look around the shelves of your local supermarket you will find foods from all over the world.

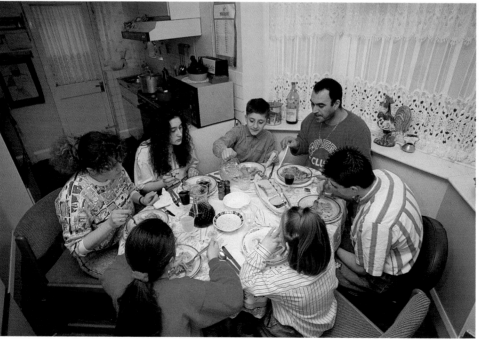

◁ Eating together is a social occasion for the whole family. It is a time when everyone can gather together and relax and talk. If you don't bother to eat properly, or just have quick snacks, you miss out on all this.

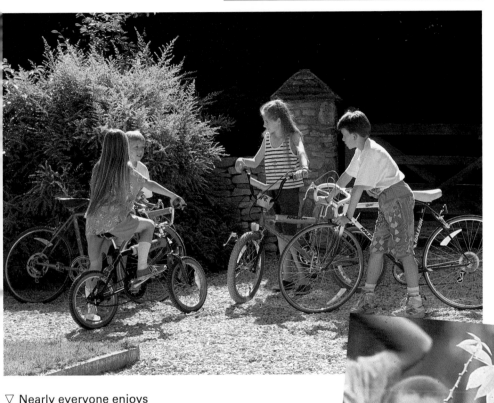

◁ Eating a good diet is not enough to ensure your good health, and getting adequate exercise is as important as diet. Cycling is excellent exercise which will give you a healthy appetite.

▽ Malnutrition and starvation affect many people in the developing, or Third World countries. There should be enough food for everyone, but, sadly, it does not always reach those who need it.

▽ Nearly everyone enjoys hamburgers but they contain lots of fat so you shouldn't eat them too often.

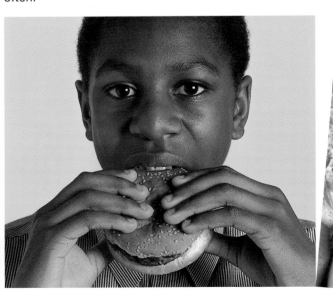

DIET AND DIGESTION

Food contains a mixture of important nutrients which all contribute towards health. The main nutrients we obtain from food are proteins, fats and carbohydrates, as well as vitamins and minerals, which are needed in much smaller amounts. These substances are taken into the body as we eat, then absorbed through the intestines during digestion.

Most food substances need to be broken down, or digested, so that they are in a form in which they can pass into the body and be used. Powerful chemicals called enzymes break down the swallowed food into a liquid, from whicn the digested nutrients are absorbed and carried in the blood to the parts of the body where they are needed.

An important use for these nutrients is to provide energy to power the body, as well as building materials for making new cells and repairing organs. Lack of some of these important nutrients, particularly in children who are growing fast, can cause some serious health problems. However, for people living in Western countries, too much food is a more likely problem, and deficiencies are not common.

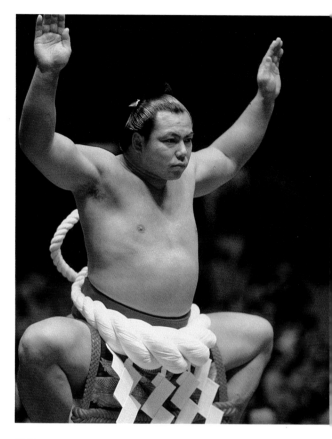

△ Japanese sumo wrestlers eat huge amounts of food to increase their weight.

▽ Vegetarian or meat-based meals can contain the proper balance of nutrients.

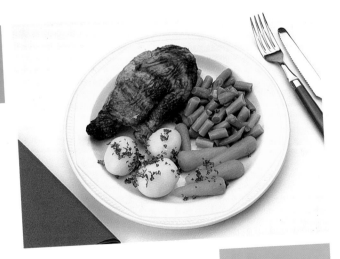

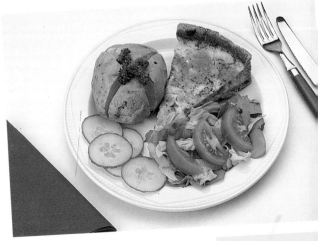

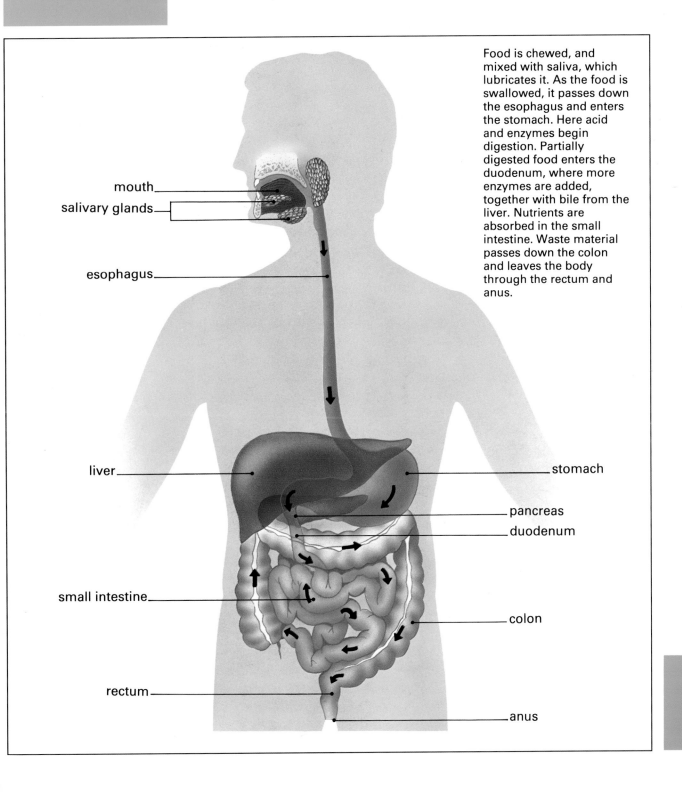

Food is chewed, and mixed with saliva, which lubricates it. As the food is swallowed, it passes down the esophagus and enters the stomach. Here acid and enzymes begin digestion. Partially digested food enters the duodenum, where more enzymes are added, together with bile from the liver. Nutrients are absorbed in the small intestine. Waste material passes down the colon and leaves the body through the rectum and anus.

mouth

salivary glands

esophagus

liver

small intestine

rectum

stomach

pancreas

duodenum

colon

anus

PROTEINS

Protein is one of the most important nutrients obtained from the diet. Every living cell in your body contains protein, and your muscles are almost completely made up of this substance. Protein can be obtained equally well from plant and animal sources. This is why a well-planned vegetarian diet can be a perfectly healthy one.

Protein molecules are very large, so they cannot be absorbed directly into the body from food. Instead, they are broken down into amino acids during digestion so that they can pass into the blood. They are then reassembled into the different types of protein required by the body.

Many important substances needed to maintain life are proteins, and these are

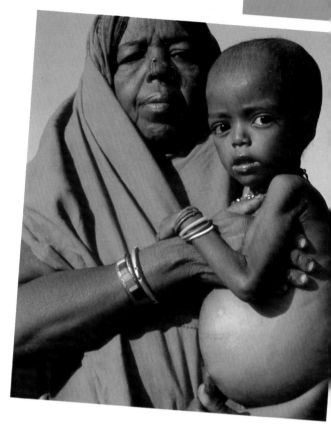

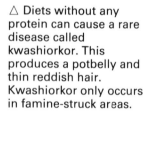

△ Diets without any protein can cause a rare disease called kwashiorkor. This produces a potbelly and thin reddish hair. Kwashiorkor only occurs in famine-struck areas.

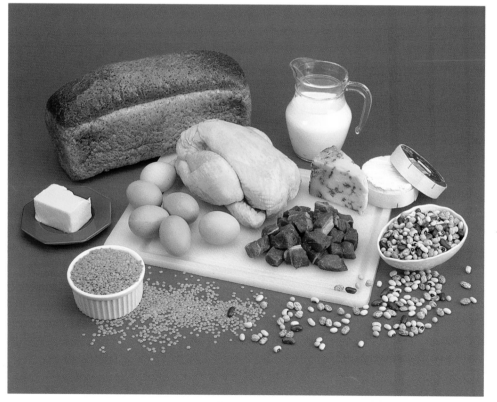

◁ Meat is a common source of protein, but this important nutrient can be obtained from many other sources. Bread, legumes, and dairy products all contain lots of protein.

constantly being produced inside living cells and poured out into the blood to be carried around the body, ready for use.

Large amounts of protein are used during growth to build muscle tissue and tissue for other parts of the body. Protein is also used to build the new cells needed to replace those that have come to the end of their useful lives. In an emergency, when your body is not receiving enough food, protein can also be used to provide energy for the body. This is a last resort however, as it means breaking down healthy tissue to release the energy stored in it.

The most common sources of protein are meat, fish, dairy products – such as milk and cheese – eggs, cereals and legumes.

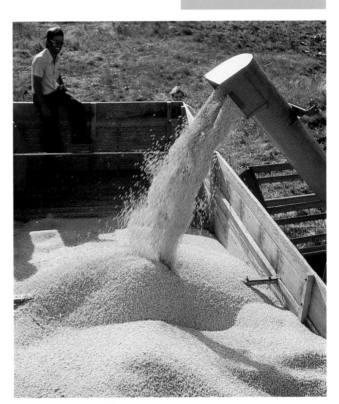

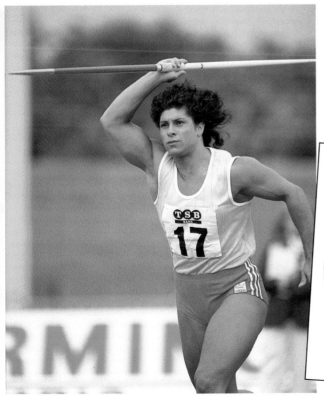

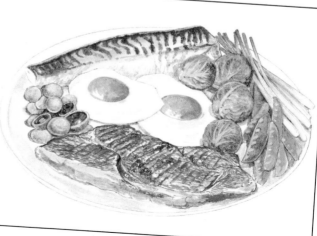

◁ ▽ Many athletes eat a special high-protein diet to build extra muscle and improve their performance.

△ The seeds of the soybean plant provide one of the world's most important sources of protein and oil.

SUGARS

Sugars are members of a group of food substances called carbohydrates, which are present in many different types of plant and vegetable foods. The simplest form of sugar, glucose, can be immediately absorbed into the body without the need for digestion. Other types of sugar, including starch, need to be broken down into smaller parts by digestion before they can be used.

Sugar gives food a pleasant, sweet taste, but its only real function in the diet is to provide energy. Sugar is broken down, or "burned," by oxygen breathed in from the air around us, releasing energy to power the chemical reactions which maintain life.

Our diets contain large amounts of sugar, and this can be a risk to health by leading to overweight and tooth decay. If we take in too much sugar, some of the energy it releases is stored as an energy reserve in the form of

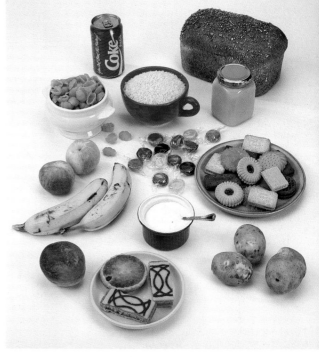

(Top right) Sugars and other carbohydrates are found in many different types of food and drink. These substances are sources of energy.

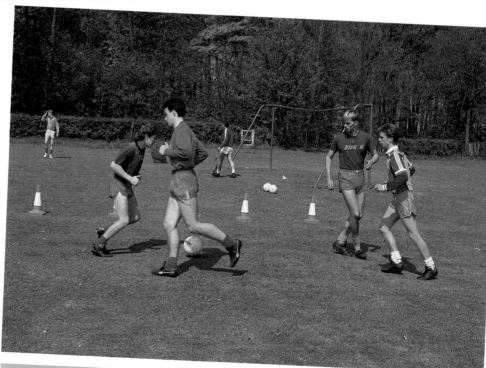

▷ Plenty of exercise is important to burn off excess energy obtained from the diet, as well as toning up the muscles.

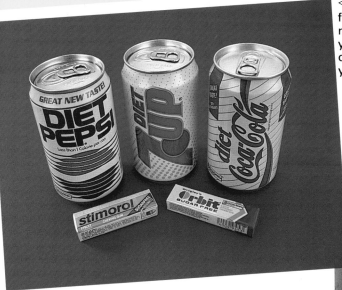

◁ You can buy many foods that contain little or no sugar. These will help you keep your weight down, and help protect your teeth.

▽ Eating too much food containing lots of carbohydrate will soon make you overweight, as well as damage your teeth.

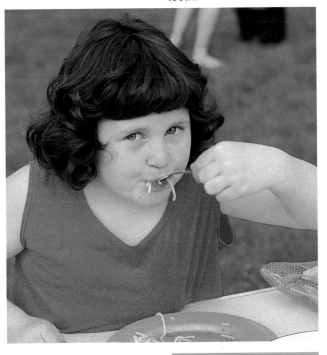

△ Tooth decay begins when bacteria, present in plaque coating the teeth, feed on sugar present in our food. The bacteria produce acid, which first softens the tooth enamel, then begins to eat into the softer dentine. Eventually the damage reaches into the pulp cavity. Bacteria attack the soft tissue, and the entire tooth decays.

fat, causing overweight. This in turn may lead to high blood pressure and heart disease later in life, and may increase the risk of other diseases, such as diabetes.

The other main risk to health is tooth decay. Bacteria living in the mouth feed on sugar and release acid which attacks the teeth, causing cavities. Too many sweet foods encourage this tooth decay.

EAT MORE FIBER!

Like sugar, fiber is a form of carbohydrate, but it cannot be digested, so it is not truly a nutrient. Fiber is a plant substance, made up mostly from the remains of plant cell walls. Its function in the diet is to bulk up the food in the intestines, keeping it soft and easily moved through the intestines until the undigested remains leave the body as feces. Some of this fiber is in solid form, while other fiber substances are sticky and may help keep the intestines healthy in other ways. One type of fiber, called soluble fiber (found in foods such as oatmeal), may also reduce the amount of fat circulating in the blood.

Eating food that is low in fiber means that most is digested, leaving only a small amount

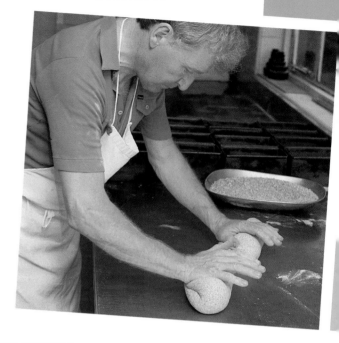

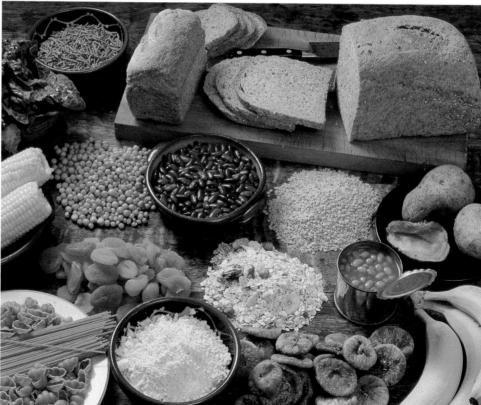

(top right) Since the value of fiber has been recognized, many more people buy whole wheat bread, which is much better for you. It contains all the fiber from the original grain.

▷ Fiber is an indigestible form of carbohydrate which helps keep the bowel healthy. There is lots of fiber in whole wheat flour and foods that are made from it. Fiber is also present in root vegetables, cereals, fruit, and legumes. It can be added to food as bran, but this does not taste pleasant and it is better to eat foods naturally rich in fiber.

of hard material that is difficult to pass along the intestines. In the process of peristalsis, the intestinal wall contracts in a series of waves that push the food along, but if the food is hard and of very small volume, the muscles have to strain very hard to shift it. This can cause constipation and piles, as well as some more unpleasant diseases.

There is plenty of fiber in fruit, vegetables and legumes (peas and beans), as well as added fiber in many breakfast cereals. Fiber is naturally present in grain, but most is removed in the form of bran in making white flour, so try to eat plenty of foods made with whole wheat flour, rather than putting bran on your food.

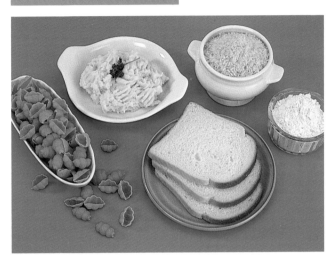

△ Foods made from refined white flour contain little fiber.

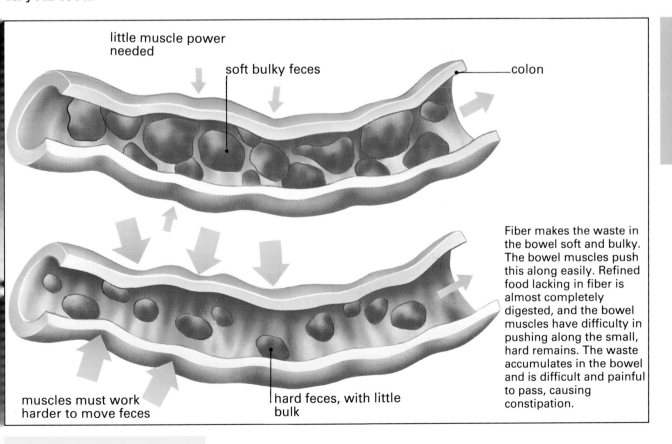

little muscle power needed

soft bulky feces

colon

muscles must work harder to move feces

hard feces, with little bulk

Fiber makes the waste in the bowel soft and bulky. The bowel muscles push this along easily. Refined food lacking in fiber is almost completely digested, and the bowel muscles have difficulty in pushing along the small, hard remains. The waste accumulates in the bowel and is difficult and painful to pass, causing constipation.

FATS

Fats are found in both animal and plant foods. Milk, meat and cooking oil are all common sources of fat – oil being a form of fat which is liquid at ordinary temperatures. Fat is most important as an energy store for the body, breaking down to release energy when it is needed. It is also required in much smaller amounts for growth and repair of the body. Fat is stored beneath the skin as insulation to keep the body warm. However, if you are eating more fat than is needed, it can also build up in some areas of the body to make you overweight.

There are several different types of fat, and they have different effects on the body. Saturated fat is mostly found in red meat, but is also present in dairy products such as butter, some vegetable oils, and other foods. In large amounts, this saturated fat causes fatty substances to be deposited on the walls

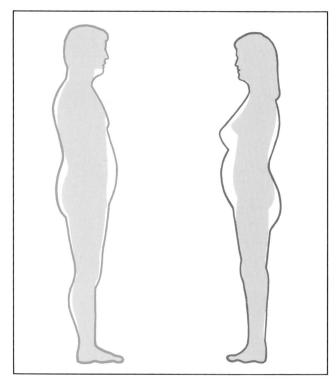

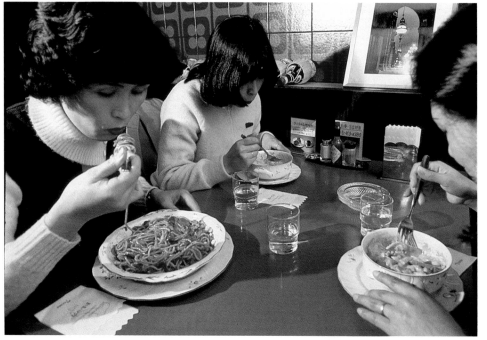

△ Fat is stored in different places in men and women. Men store most fat in the abdomen and around the neck, while women have a thin layer of insulating fat over most of the body. Women also store fat in their breasts, buttocks and thighs.

◁ The Japanese diet contains little meat, and for this reason, contains only a small amount of saturated fat. Heart disease, which is associated with high levels of saturated fat in the diet, is uncommon in Japan. In addition, their low fat, mainly vegetarian diet, contains fewer calories than our own, so overweight is less common.

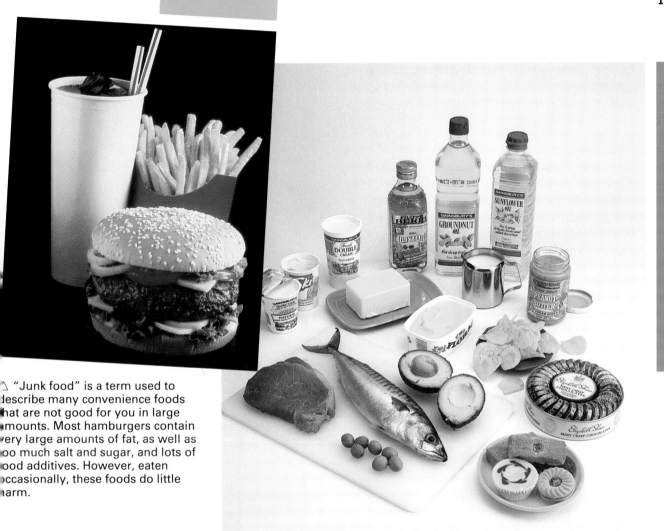

△ "Junk food" is a term used to describe many convenience foods that are not good for you in large amounts. Most hamburgers contain very large amounts of fat, as well as too much salt and sugar, and lots of food additives. However, eaten occasionally, these foods do little harm.

of blood vessels, gradually making them narrower and obstructing the flow of blood. These deposits can eventually lead to heart disease, strokes, and other illnesses. In countries where little animal (saturated) fat is eaten, such diseases are uncommon.

Polyunsaturated and monounsaturated fats have a different makeup to saturated fats and are less likely to cause heart disease. They are found in olive oil, sunflower oil, some nuts and vegetables, and oily fish, such as salmon and mackerel.

△ Many foods contain fat, and sometimes this is hidden. For example, potato chips contain lots of fat, and so do avocados (very unusual for a fruit). Fat is always present in meat, even though the visible part can be trimmed off. Not all these fats are saturated and harmful. Fish oils and olive oil are particularly good for the heart and circulation.

BODY CHEMISTRY

Vitamins play a vital part in helping the chemical reactions of life. Most of them are needed in very small amounts, so a normal mixed diet contains all the vitamins you need. Vitamin pills are very popular, but in the West true vitamin deficiency is extremely rare, except in the very young or elderly, pregnant women, or some people eating certain ethnic or extreme vegetarian diets.

Vitamin D deficiency may affect some vegetarians, or people living on large amounts of rice. The body normally makes this vitamin in the skin, when it is exposed to sunlight, so plenty of outdoor activity will make sure that you don't experience this problem. Serious vitamin D deficiency can lead to a condition known as rickets.

Minerals are simple chemical substances needed during growth and throughout life. Calcium and phosphorus are minerals

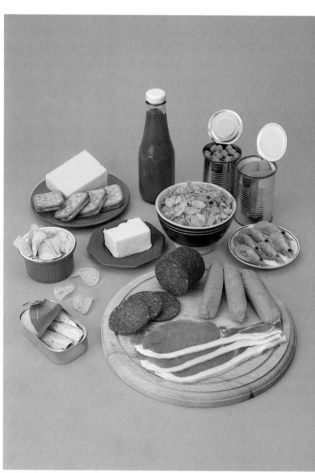

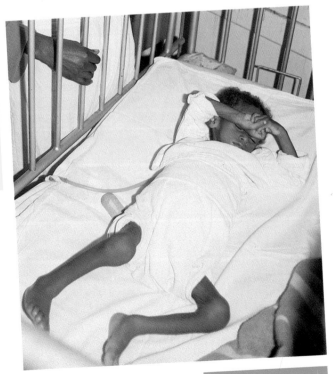

◁ Rickets is a bone disease caused by a lack of vitamin D. It keeps the bones of children from hardening properly, so they become permanently bent and the joints are damaged. Rickets is rare in people who eat a good, balanced diet and get plenty of fresh air and sunlight.

△ Salt is added to many foods to improve their taste, and to act as a preservative. We take in much more salt than we need, and this could be harmful later in life. Snack foods, like potato chips and salted nuts, have extremely high salt levels, and so do preserved meats like bacon salami and sausage.

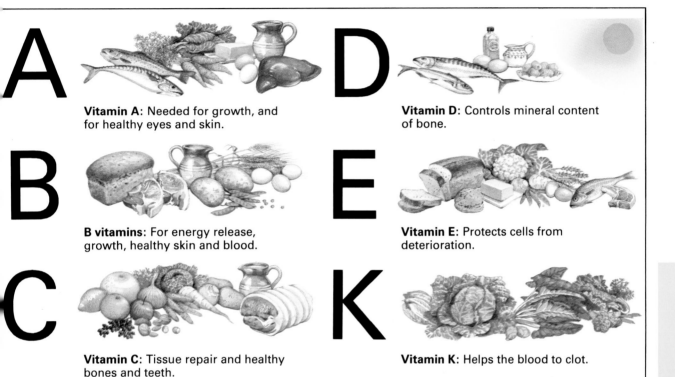

Vitamin A: Needed for growth, and for healthy eyes and skin.

B vitamins: For energy release, growth, healthy skin and blood.

Vitamin C: Tissue repair and healthy bones and teeth.

Vitamin D: Controls mineral content of bone.

Vitamin E: Protects cells from deterioration.

Vitamin K: Helps the blood to clot.

Fresh food contains lots of vitamins, but some are destroyed by cooking.

▷ Milk contains lots of calcium, a mineral which you need for healthy bones and teeth.

needed for bone growth, and iron and sodium are needed for healthy blood. Salt contains sodium, and this is the most common chemical in the body. We take in more salt in our diets than we need, and it may cause health problems. Mineral supplements are seldom necessary, except for pregnant women, to cope with the needs of the developing baby. Iron deficiency is common during pregnancy and can lead to anemia.

Minerals are present in large amounts in vegetables, but they can be washed out by boiling them for too long. Light boiling or steaming retains these minerals much better.

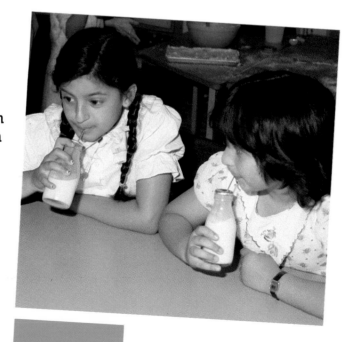

ADDITIVES

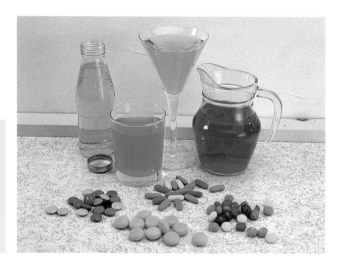

△ Artificial colorings are added to many candies and drinks to make them more attractive. All of these coloring substances have been tested to prove their safety, but some people fear that there could be risks when they are eaten over a long period of time, so they try to avoid colorings and other additives.

Food additives are used for many different reasons. They may be colorings used to make food look better, they can add flavor, and they can preserve food or improve its texture in various ways. All of these additives must be listed on the labels of foods and drinks. Some people are concerned that additives could be a health risk, and prefer to buy additive-free foods. It is known that rarely, some people react to particular additives, in which case they have to check food labels carefully to confirm that the food is safe for them to eat. However, additives are not a serious health risk as so few people suffer in this way.

Some additives are essential because they prevent the growth of dangerous bacteria. Many meat products such as sausages and pies would be unsafe without some

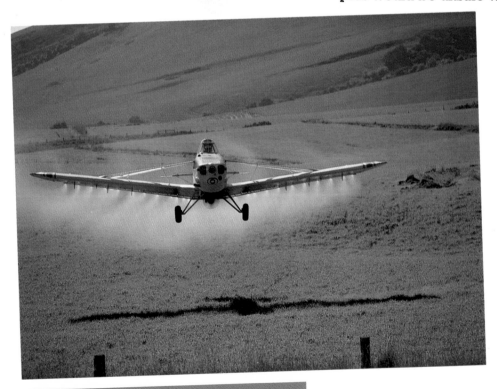

◁ In large farms all around the world, chemical fertilizers and pesticides are sprayed on crops and pastures to improve their growth. There are fears that these chemicals could get into water supplies and be harmful to people drinking the water. Also, even after washing sprayed fruit or vegetables, some of the chemicals will remain and may be harmful.

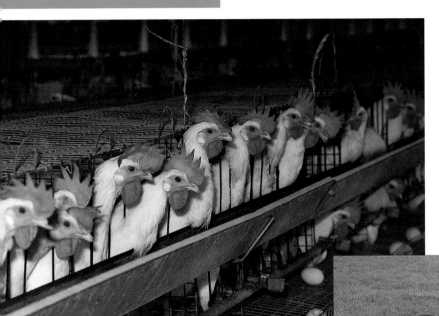

◁ Many farm animals must receive drugs regularly to keep healthy. These battery chickens would quickly die of infection if they were not treated, as their conditions are unhygienic. Sometimes the drugs find their way into meat or eggs, causing a risk that our own bacteria could become used to the drugs used. Salmonella may infect poultry and eggs, and can cause serious food poisoning. Many people prefer to eat eggs and meat from animals that have not been treated with drugs, like these free-range pigs *(below)*.

▽ Organic foods are produced without the help of chemical fertilizers or pesticides. This may mean that they are less attractive than conventional foods, and perhaps more expensive because fewer healthy crops can be produced. Many people still prefer to buy them to avoid any possible health risk.

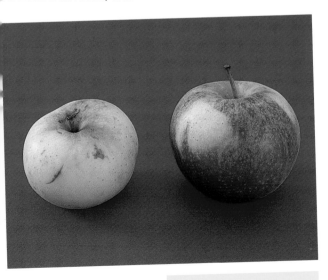

preservatives. Colorings and flavorings are not essential, so you may choose to avoid foods to which they have been added.

Other "hidden" substances in food are the remains of chemical treatments given to animals or crops mainly to improve growth and prevent disease. These can be drugs, fertilizers, or pesticides used to kill insects and plant diseases. There are many regulations to ensure that these substances are present in only very small amounts, but it is wise to wash fruit and vegetables thoroughly before they are used.

FOOD HYGIENE

Bacteria and other microscopic organisms swarm in the air and the environment. They can live and grow on any type of food, and may cause infections when the food is eaten. They also produce very poisonous substances called toxins which make people extremely ill. Food poisoning occurs when this contaminated food is eaten, causing diarrhea and vomiting.

To prevent food contamination, careful hygiene is needed in handling and storing food. So, people with boils or cuts on their hands should never handle food, in case bacteria are spread. Many foods must be stored in a refrigerator or freezer, where the

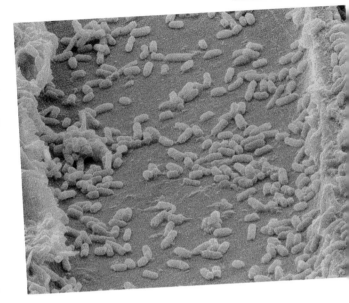

◁ Careful kitchen food hygiene is essential, particularly in restaurants.

△ These Salmonella bacteria are growing on a kitchen cutting board.

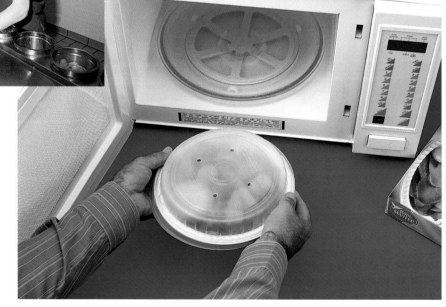

▷ Microwave cooking is very useful because it allows food to be heated very rapidly. A microwave oven can also be used to defrost frozen foods quickly. However, it must be used carefully, because it does not heat the food evenly, and there will be "cold spots." This means that frozen foods may not defrost properly, and when cooking, parts of the food may not get hot enough to kill all the bacteria present. Even heating is important when reheating foods, and when cooking poultry, which may contain Salmonella.

low temperatures slow down or prevent the growth of bacteria.

However carefully the food is handled there will always be a few bacteria present. Proper cooking destroys most of the bacteria, but if toxins are already present, they will still remain after cooking and can cause illness. It is very important to thaw frozen foods properly, and to cook them thoroughly, especially when using microwave ovens which may leave "cold spots" where bacteria could survive.

Most prepared foods today have "sell by" or "use by" dates on the label, which must be strictly followed.

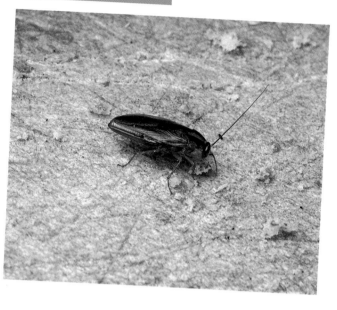

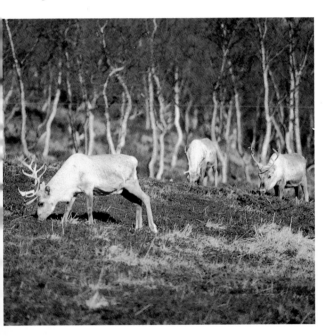

△ Cockroaches are large insects which thrive in warm, damp places such as kitchens. Cockroaches carry bacteria and are a serious health risk.

▽ Because radiation can kill bacteria, it can be used in low doses to sterilize and preserve food in sealed packages, so it need not be refrigerated.

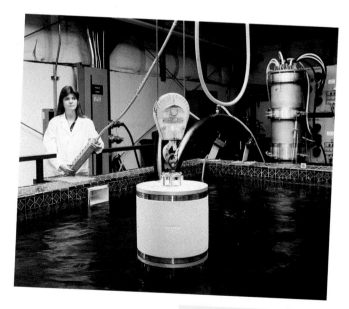

△ When the Chernobyl atomic reactor in Russia released huge amounts of radiation into the atmosphere, clouds of radioactive dust traveled as far as Lapland. The radioactive material was absorbed by moss which, when eaten by reindeer, made them dangerous to eat. Some radiation also reached Britain, and lambs from some mountainous areas were banned from being sold for meat.

STOMACH UPSETS

Many people pick up a stomach virus when they go on vacation or visit other countries. Our bodies usually become accustomed to the food bacteria most common around our homes, so we are not made sick by them. But when we go away, we encounter types which the body has not learned to cope with, so they can cause sickness and diarrhea. There are other reasons for this increased risk of food infections. In hotter climates, bacteria grow very rapidly, and standards of hygiene may not be as high as those we are used to. This also applies to drinking water, which is sometimes dangerous to drink because it contains bacteria which do not bother the local people.

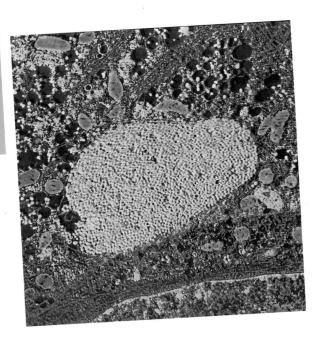

△ This yellow mass contains hundreds of virus particles, of a type which often causes diarrhea and vomiting.

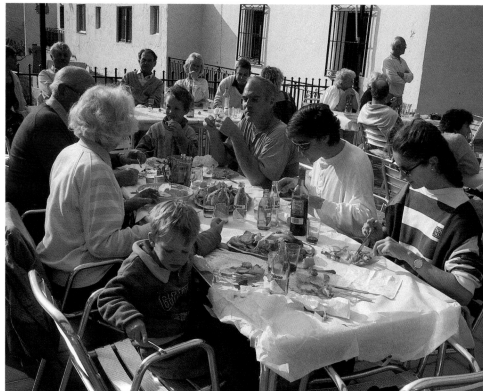

▷ Eating foreign meals in warmer climates often causes a stomach virus or diarrhea. This is because we are not used to the common bacteria which do not trouble the local people.

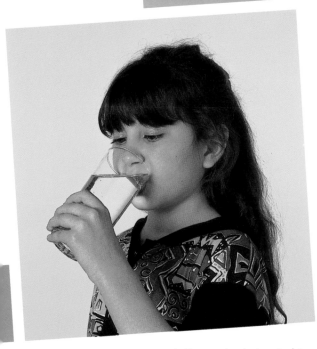

△ Tap water is treated to make it safe to drink. In many parts of the world, tap water is contaminated and must be boiled before it is used.

Vomiting and diarrhea are the body's way of trying to rid itself of contaminated food or drink. The muscles around the abdomen contract sharply to squeeze the stomach contents up and out through the mouth, causing vomiting. In diarrhea, the muscles around the intestines work rapidly to pass the contaminated food through as fast as possible. It is ejected from the body in a liquid form, because the intestines have not had time to solidify the material into feces.

Gas is caused by swallowing air, usually during eating, in which case it may be "burped" up from the stomach. Gas is also produced by the action of bacteria on some types of food in the intestine, and leaves the body through the anus.

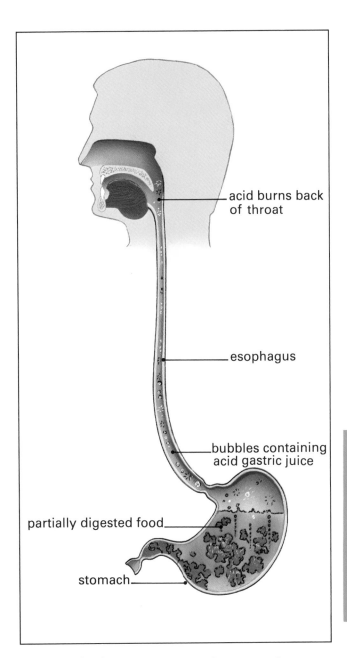

acid burns back of throat

esophagus

bubbles containing acid gastric juice

partially digested food

stomach

△ Indigestion is a stomach pain which may follow eating. It may mean that you have swallowed a lot of air while chewing and swallowing food, which bubbles up the esophagus, causing "burping," and sometimes bringing acid stomach contents up into the throat. It may also be caused by spicy foods or unripe fruit.

EATING DISORDERS

Overweight is one of the most common health problems we have in Western countries, and most of us could be just as healthy if we lost a few pounds. But some people put on so much weight that their whole system is under a considerable strain. This condition of obesity means that exercise is an effort, you become breathless, and there is a strain on your heart and circulation even while you are still young. If you are so overweight that it is worrying you, ask your doctor for advice. A change in diet could keep you healthier and feeling better.

Some people have the reverse problem. They feel that they are overweight, even though they are actually perfectly normal.

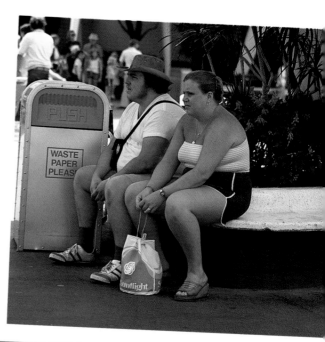

△ Overweight is very common in people living in Western countries, where most of us eat too much food, often of the wrong type. Overweight may start in children, and as they grow into adults, it will eventually affect their health.

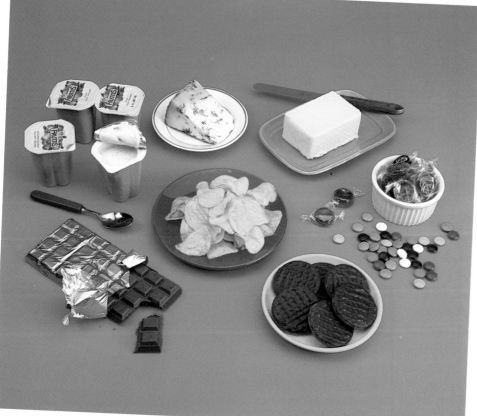

◁ Foods that contain lots of sugar and fat will make you fat if you eat a lot of them. By finding out what should be in a healthy diet, you will know which types of foods to avoid. Look for low fat, low sugar content foods to help prevent a weight and health problem.

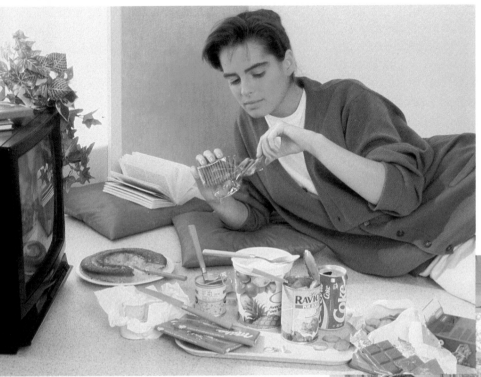

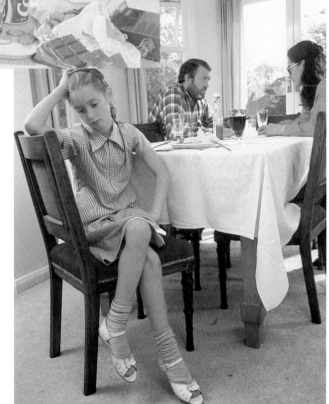

◁ Bulimia nervosa causes people to often eat large amounts of food. Then, because they fear putting on weight, they will force themselves to vomit before the food can be digested. (This is a set up picture and the model shown is not suffering from bulimia nervosa.)

▷ Anorexia is a disease in which young people believe that they are fat, and therefore eat as little as possible. This makes them painfully thin, and some anorexics become very ill. This is a serious emotional disorder, which needs special treatment.

People with anorexia nervosa, which usually affects adolescents, have a fear of overweight, so they starve themselves, often pretending to eat or hiding their food. Eventually they become starved and extremely ill. In a related condition called bulimia nervosa, they eat normally, or even more than normal, then force themselves to vomit before the food can be digested. Both of these conditions have emotional causes, and because they can be very serious if left untreated, it is important to discuss any such problem with your doctor, whether it affects yourself, or someone you know.

SPECIAL DIETS

Vegetarian diets can be very healthy, but some more specialized forms of vegetarian diet need particular care if you are to remain healthy. Vegans for example, eat only food of plant origin, with no meat or dairy products at all. In order to stay healthy on such a diet, it is often necessary to take vitamin supplements.

Several types of Asian diets are very healthy, being low in fat and high in carbohydrates. These diets are often largely vegetarian, either for religious reasons or from custom. There are several other types of diet eaten for religious reasons. Muslims may eat only Halal meat, and some Jews eat only kosher food. This means that their meat has to be prepared according to strict religious rules, and there are several items of food which are completely forbidden.

People with diabetes need special diets in which the amount of sugar is carefully controlled. Other people cannot tolerate a substance called gluten, present in certain types of cereal. They need to eat a special gluten-free diet if they are to remain healthy.

Some people are sensitive or even allergic to certain foods, which can make them ill. Eggs and sometimes milk are thought to cause an allergic reaction in some babies and adults. Eating strawberries, shellfish and nuts makes some people develop an itchy rash called urticaria.

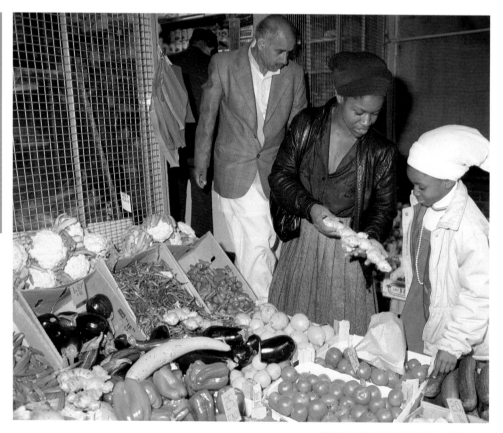

◁ Rastafarians belong to a West Indian religious sect who do not eat fruit or vegetables that have been treated with fertilizers or pesticides.

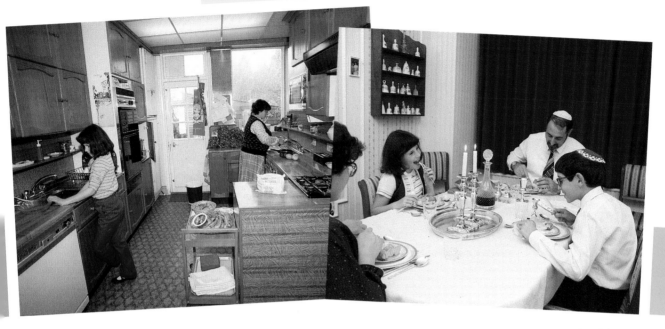

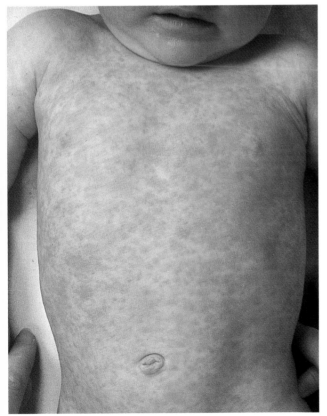

◁ This skin rash, or urticaria, is an allergic reaction, that some people experience when they eat strawberries. ▽ It can also be caused by eating shellfish or nuts.

△ For many Jewish families, mealtimes are religious occasions. Meat and dairy products are kept separate, according to religious rules.

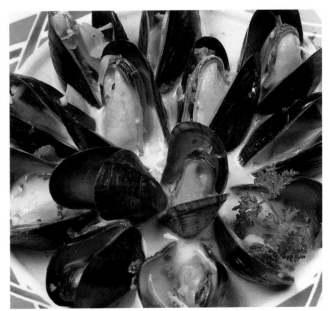

SENSIBLE EATING

Because eating a poor or unbalanced diet is known to be a serious health risk, there are now several important recommendations for improving our diets, and our health. These are:

● Eat *less* sugar, to control excess weight.

● Eat *less* salt, to help avoid diseases such as high blood pressure.

● Eat *less* fat to keep weight under control. In particular, cut down on saturated fat.

● Eat *more* fiber to keep the intestines healthy.

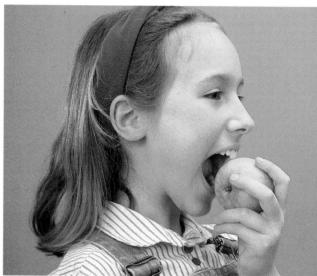

△ Sensible eating means cutting out many high calorie snacks. "An apple a day" is a good alternative to candy or cookies, and it won't have such a bad effect on your teeth or weight. Nuts and dried fruit are also useful and healthy snacks.

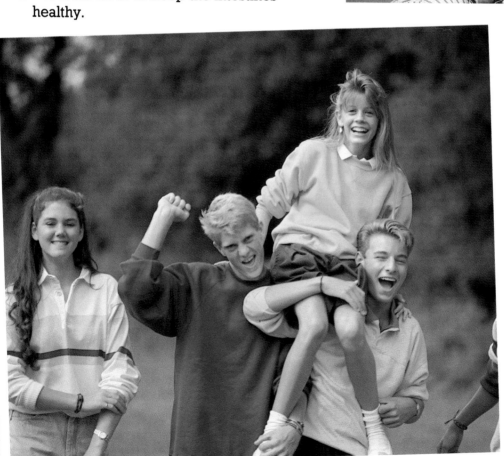

◁ Positive health practice means that you will feel good. Eating the right kind of diet in the proper amounts, and taking adequate exercise to keep your circulation and muscles healthy, all combine to make you feel and perform at your peak.

FAST RUNNING		650 Calories per hour
SWIMMING		500 Calories per hour
FOOTBALL		400 Calories per hour
CYCLING		300 Calories per hour
DANCING		250 Calories per hour
READING		100 Calories per hour
SLEEPING		65 Calories per hour

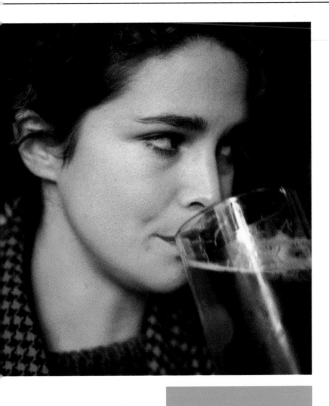

◁ Many people do not realize that alcohol contains large amounts of calories. This means that people who drink a lot usually get fat, even though they may be careful about what they eat.

△ When we switch from resting to running, our energy usage increases 10 times, from 65 to 650 Calories per hour. This makes it obvious why too much inactivity can cause you to become fat.

Eating a sensible diet and exercising should keep your weight at the proper level for your age. Dieting is definitely not a good idea while you are still growing, unless this is under the supervision of your doctor, for some medical reason. It is relatively easy to cut out sugar and sweet foods like cake, but you should remember that sugar and other nutrients are "hidden" in many foods. For example, crackers contain lots of salt, and most baked beans contain added sugar. It is sensible to get used to reading food labels so that you know what you are eating.

MORE INFORMATION

Growth is not a steady process, and at some times of life, you will notice that you are getting taller or heavier, because you grow out of your clothes. You grow fastest during the first three years, and then slow down, but will grow quickly again during your teens. It is during these growth spurts that you need most food energy, in the form of Calories.

Children use the following Calories per day:		
Age	Sex	Cal
9-11	both sexes	2200
12-14	boys	2650
	girls	2150
15-17	boys	2900
	girls	2150

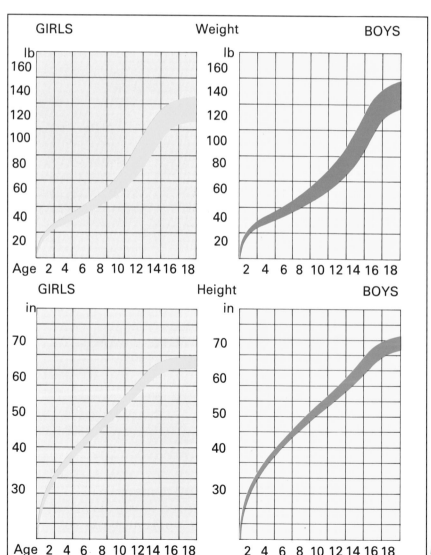

These graphs show that girls and boys grow at different rates, especially in their late teens. They therefore need different amounts of food per day.

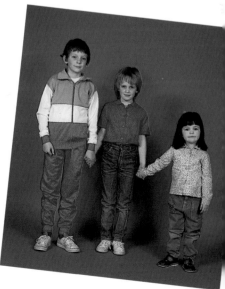

GLOSSARY

Additive: A substance added to food to improve its flavor or appearance, to preserve it, or to change it in some other way. Some people believe that additives may be harmful.

Amino acid: Family of related substances that are produced by the digestion of proteins. They are built up again into different proteins inside the body.

Calcium: Mineral substance obtained from food, which forms the hard tissue in bones and teeth. Also important in nerve and muscle activity.

Carbohydrate: Food substance containing hydrogen, oxygen and carbon. Sugars, starches and fiber are all carbohydrates. Sugars and starches are broken down to provide energy.

Digestion: The process in which the body breaks down food to produce substances that can be absorbed into the body and used.

Enzyme: Substance produced by digestive glands, which helps in the breakdown of foods during digestion. Other enzymes take part in cell processes.

Fat: Substance used mainly as an energy store. Fat is deposited in the body when too many calories are present in the diet.

Fiber: Form of carbohydrate present in unrefined vegetable and cereal foods, which cannot be digested. Fiber is important for the health of the bowel.

Glucose: Form of sugar that can be rapidly broken down to provide energy when needed.

Iron: Mineral substance obtained from green vegetables, liver and kidney, which is important in the formation of red blood cells.

Nutrient: Substance produced by the process of digestion which can be used by the body to provide energy, and to grow and repair new tissues and cells.

Polyunsaturated fats: Form of fat which is associated with a reduced risk of heart disease. Many vegetable fats and oils are of this type.

Protein: Important food substance which is used in the body to build muscle and other tissues. In digestion, protein is broken down into amino acids, so these can be absorbed. Protein is present in meat and dairy products, cereal, nuts and many other foods.

Saturated fat: Form of fat which may cause fatty deposits in the walls of blood vessels, and can lead to heart disease if there is too much in the diet. Saturated fats and oils are present in large amounts in meat and dairy products, and in some vegetable fats and oils. Diets high in saturated fat are considered a health risk.

Sodium: The most plentiful substance in the body; most of this sodium is present in the form of sodium chloride, or common salt. This helps to maintain a constant environment in the fluid which bathes all the body cells. Too much sodium in the diet could be a health risk for people with high blood pressure.

Starch: Form of carbohydrate which is broken down into sugar in the process of digestion. Starch is present in large amounts in cereals and vegetables.

Vitamin: Substance obtained from the diet, which helps in many chemical reactions in the body. Most vitamins are needed in only very small amounts, and vitamin supplements are not normally necessary.

INDEX

PRINTED IN BELGIUM BY
proost
INTERNATIONAL BOOK PRODUCTION